Gastric Sleeve

*The Practical Gastric Sleeve
Surgery Handbook for Optimal
Weight Loss Results*

by

Michael Beck

© Copyright 2017 by Michael Beck
All rights reserved.

information in question by the reader will render any resulting actions solely under their purview. There are no scenarios in which the publisher or the original author of this work can be in any fashion deemed liable for any hardship or damages that may befall them after undertaking information described herein.

Additionally, the information in the following pages is intended only for informational purposes and should thus be thought of as universal. As befitting its nature, it is presented without assurance regarding its prolonged validity or interim quality. Trademarks that are mentioned are done without written consent and can in no way be considered an endorsement from the trademark holder.

Table of Contents

Introduction

Congratulations on downloading this book and thank you for doing so.

The following chapters will discuss some of the different things that you should know about gastric sleeve surgery. Many people today are suffering from obesity and they have a lot of trouble trying to lose weight. While the gastric sleeve is not a miracle method to help you out (you will have to put in some of the work to see results), it can be a great tool to get you started. This guidebook is going to talk about the gastric sleeve and will answer some of your pressing questions about what goes on before, during, and after the surgery.

We will start out this guidebook by talking about what the gastric sleeve is and some of the benefits that come with getting this kind of surgery. We will then move on to some of the questions that you should ask your doctor before getting this surgery as well as talking about the diets that you will have to follow before, during, and after the surgery to really see results. This guidebook will end with some information about stomach stretching as well as some tips that will help you to be successful.

Gastric sleeve surgery is not an option that you should enter into lightly. You do need to take a step up and be willing to change your lifestyle and diet habits for this surgery to be successful over the long term. But if you have dedicated yourself to making these changes and work hard afterward, you are sure to get the results that you want.

There are plenty of books on this subject on the market, thanks again for choosing this one! Every effort was made to ensure it is full of as much useful information as possible, please enjoy!

Chapter 1: What is Gastric Sleeve Surgery?

There are many people in our country who are looking to lose weight. They are tired of being overweight and they may be dealing with some intense health problems that will not go away until the weight is all gone. These people have probably tried to lose weight for a long time, trying out a lot of the different meal plans that are on the market and even some of the fad options, with no results. They either barely lose any weight or they will lose some weight before gaining it and more back.

This can be really frustrating for most people to handle. They feel that they are putting in all of the work that is necessary without getting any of the results. The gastric sleeve is sometimes one of the last options that they have left before their health conditions get even more serious.

This surgery is not something that you just get on a whim, though. There have to be some serious changes for the patient because going back on the old diet and habits will just make you gain all of the weight back. There is also a significant amount of pain and sums of money for this surgery; so, it is not a decision to be taken lightly. Patients would have to spend time discussing the options with their doctor and finding a nutritionist to work with. But for those who have tried everything else, it can be the right option for them.

Restrictive operations, like what happens with gastric sleeve surgery, are used in order to help people lose weight because the surgery will make the stomach smaller. When the stomach becomes smaller, you become fuller with less food and you can take in fewer calories. You will need to make some changes for the rest of your life, such as eating smaller portion sizes and making sure that you eat foods that are high in nutrients if you want to continue to see the weight loss.

When you and your doctor decide to go ahead with this surgery, the surgery itself is pretty easy to accomplish. The surgeon is going to make a big incision into your abdomen in an open procedure or they can do a few smaller incisions with a small instrument and a camera, which is the laparoscopic approach. Most doctors prefer the latter because it has a quicker healing time and it will not cause as much pain to the patient.

After the incisions are made, half of your stomach or more will be removed, which is going to leave a tube or a vertical sleeve that looks to be about half the size of a banana. Then the surgeon will use some surgical staples to help close up your new stomach. It is important to remember that in this kind of surgery, part of the stomach is removed so you will not be able to reverse this kind of surgery.

In some cases, this surgery is going to be the primary step to helping you to lose weight and other times it will be just part of a larger approach to help with that weight loss. For example, if you are going to have a duodenal switch surgery but you still have a lot of weight to lose first, you may find that a gastric sleeve surgery can be what you need to help with this.

After the surgery is done, you are going to have some pain in your stomach and it is possible that you will be on pain medication for a week or more afterward. The doctor did cut into your stomach and so this can be a bit sore and tender. You will also notice that you will feel full more quickly after eating meals (even though you will be on a mostly liquid diet for the first while after operation). In some cases, your food may end up emptying into the small intestine too fast in what is known as dumping syndrome. If this does happen, it can cause diarrhea and you may feel sick, shaky, and faint. If you are not careful with the nutrients that you are taking in, these smaller meals may leave you lacking in the vitamins and nutrients that you receive.

Depending on the method that the doctor used to perform the surgery, whether they did the laparoscopic or the open option, you will need to watch your level of activity after the operation. If you had the open surgery, you will need to avoid a lot of exercise or heavy lifting during the time of recovery so that you can give the stomach some time to heal. You probably won't be able to get back to your normal routine for about a month or so when this happens. The recovery time for the laparoscopic procedure is going to be a lot faster, which is one reason that a lot of surgeons like to go with it.

While we are going to spend some time talking about the foods that you are allowed to eat with this surgery, you will also need to follow the instructions that your doctor gives to you. In the first month, once the operation is done, your stomach is going to be really sensitive. This means that it will only be able to handle a little bit of very soft foods and some liquids while it continues to heal. You must remember to sip water throughout the day so that you won't become dehydrated in the process.

Right after you have the operation, your bowel movements are not going to be as regular as you were used to in the past. This is pretty common. You should work to avoid constipation as much as possible and try not to strain too much with your bowel movements.

Over time, and with the approval of your doctor, you will start to add those solid foods back into the diet. Make sure that you carefully chew all of the food that you eat and eat slowly so that you know when you feel full. This is something that takes patients some time to learn because you will end up eating a lot less food than you did before.

If you end up not completely chewing your food, or you do not stop eating at the right time, you are going to feel uncomfortable and sometimes you may get sick. If you are not careful with the types of drinks that you consume, such as choosing to go with soda and fruit juice, you may find that it is hard to lose weight. If you are not able to keep your portion sizes small, your stomach can start to stretch out and you will not see the benefits that you want from this surgery.

For the most part, you will need to work with a dietician or a nutritionist to help you come up with a game plan for your dietary needs after the surgery is done. They are going to help you learn about proper portion control, help you to make sure that you pick out meals that have the right kinds of nutrients, and will answer any questions that you may have. In some cases, even with a good diet plan in place, you will need to take some supplements to help ensure that you are getting the nutrients that the body needs.

Now, we have spent some time talking about the gastric sleeve surgery and how it is done, but you may wonder why some people choose to have this surgery. This kind of weight loss surgery is going to be a good choice for those who are severely overweight and those who have not been able to use medicine, exercise, or diet to help them lose the weight.

These types of surgeries are not going to be done for a few vanity pounds. For the most part, they will not be considered until the person has a body mass index that is over 40. In a few select cases, those who have a BMI that is 35 or higher and who are dealing with a life-threatening problem because of their weight may be able to get the surgeries as well.

Before you go in and try to get this surgery, it is important to think of this surgery as a tool that is going to help you to lose weight. It is not going to do all of the work for you and it is not really an instant fix. You have to make sure that you put in the work as well, getting enough exercise and eating a diet that is nice and healthy. If you are able to do these things, the gastric sleeve surgery can help you to reach your weight goal and will even prevent you from gaining the weight back.

There has been some research done to see how well the gastric sleeve is able to work. Research has shown how those who got the gastric sleeve done would lose over half of the excess weight they are holding onto. For those who have realistic expectations about how much weight they will lose, who listen to their nutritionists, and who don't miss out on appointments are more likely to see good results and to lose more weight. Of course, staying on your eating plan and being active, rather than falling back into your old habits, can help as well.

There are a few risks that can come from going with the gastric sleeve. You have to remember that it is a type of surgery so there are always those complications that you need to worry about. Sticking to the diet plan that you are given at this time is really important. It is less about the weight loss at this time (even though you will lose weight on a mostly liquid diet), and more about making sure that the stomach heals properly and doesn't become too irritated. You also need to limit your physical activity so you don't harm yourself during recovery.

Another issue that you may deal with is poor nutrition. There will be some vitamins and minerals that don't absorb well in the body because you took out a large part of your stomach. This is part of why you will work with a nutritionist. This allows you to learn how to eat the healthiest meals possible so that you get lots of nutrition to stay healthy. Most people who get this surgery will end up needing to take a multivitamin as well to help with this.

There are a few things to consider before you decide to go with a gastric sleeve. You have to remember that this is not a get quick slim option. It is not a cosmetic surgery and it will not remove any of the fatty tissue that is on the body. You will lose weight and much faster than you did in the past, but it will not instantly take the fat off.

There are many times that the gastric sleeve is going to help out those who are severely overweight (with BMI's over 40). It has been shown to help prevent heart diseases, cancer, and diabetes in those who are obese and got the surgery compared to those who didn't get the surgery.

Why should I consider this surgery?

If you are overweight and looking for a way that will help you to lose weight when the other options have failed you, you have probably looked at a wide variety of options to see what will work. There are actually a few different treatments for weight loss, so why is the gastric sleeve surgery so much better than some of the other weight loss surgeries that are out there? Some of the reasons that you would want to choose the gastric sleeve for weight loss compared to using a bypass or another option include:

- You won't have to worry about getting a medical implant like you would with gastric banding.
- You will not have to worry about an intestinal bypass like what happens with a gastric bypass.
- For those who are dealing with severe medical issues or a high BMI, this surgery is one of the safest ones for weight loss.
- This surgery is safe even in patients who have lower BMI's that are between 30 to 55.

Of course, before you decide to go through with this or any other weight loss surgery, you need to make sure that you discuss this with your doctor. If you are obese and you have gone through all of the other weight loss options, a surgical solution can be the right one for you. Your surgeon will be able to tell if you are a good candidate for this kind of surgery and will be able to discuss some of the options with you or answer any of your questions.

Advantages of this kind of surgery

It is important that you know all of the advantages that come with this kind of surgery. Some people are so excited about the idea of losing weight, but it is important to remember that you are still going through a surgery so weighing the benefits and the negatives are so important. There are a lot of great benefits that come with the gastric sleeve surgery including:

- This is a great option for helping you to lose weight. You do need to change up some of your dietary habits and activity levels after the surgery, but it is very safe and effective.
- It can help you to limit your food ingestion so that you end up eating less over time.
- It will reduce how hungry you feel and since the stomach is smaller, you will feel full faster.
- Digestion will still occur naturally and you won't have any changes in vitamin and mineral absorption.
- It will not cause dumping syndrome because you will still be using the natural outlets in the stomach.
- This will not cause food to get stuck when it enters the stomach and outside of it during the recovery period, you will not have to worry about restricting the foods you can eat.
- It is safer and has less complexity compared to other similar surgeries. There will not be any alteration or cutting of the intestines.

- It will not include adding in a medical device to the body like what happens with the gastric band.
- Even on patients who are severely obese, this surgery can be done laparoscopically. This is a much safer procedure that is easier to do and will speed up the recovery time.
- Sometimes a patient is disqualified from other surgeries for weight loss because of their medical issues or other health problems. This is not true when it comes to the gastric sleeve.
- This procedure can be used as part of a larger procedure. Sometimes it is used first to help a patient to lose weight before they go to a gastric bypass or a duodenal switch if they need more weight loss later on.
- There is also a revision option for some gastric band patients.

As you can see, there are quite a few benefits that come with using the gastric sleeve surgery. It is easy to use, doesn't have as many risks that come with some of the other weight loss surgeries, and can be very effective in helping people lose weight.

Risks of this surgery

This is a type of surgery that you are going through. You will have a doctor who is cutting into you and making your stomach smaller. While it is a more effective and safe option compared to some of the other options for weight loss, it is important to realize that there are some risks. Some of the risks that come with this kind of surgery include:

- Pain: when you are done with this surgery, you are going to end up with a lot of pain. It may take a few days before you can do much besides just sit back and recover. It will then take a few more weeks before you can get into a regular exercise routine or do anything that is too strenuous. Make sure that you take things slowly. It is much better to go slowly rather than hurting yourself or causing more complications.
- Leaking food: if you go off your diet too quickly, you could end up with food that leaks out of your stomach. Your doctor will check for this right after the surgery to make sure that this isn't a problem before you go home, but take things slowly to ensure it doesn't happen when you get home. This can cause infections or even another surgery if you are not careful.
- Stretching out the stomach: while it is fine to eat a big meal on occasion, you do need to make sure that you are careful not to eat too much for each meal, and not to snack too much in between meals, once the surgery is done. It is possible for your stomach to stretch out again after the surgery. And if the stomach stretches

out again, you could end up gaining back all of the weight that you have lost. The gastric sleeve can be a permanent solution, but you have to keep up your end of the work as well.

- Nutrient deficiency: some people forget that they are eating a lot less food than before, which means that you could end up losing out on some of the nutrients that your body needs to function properly. Your nutritionist will help you to make sure that you are getting as many nutrients as you possibly can into your diet plan, but make sure that you take in a multivitamin as well to help you stay healthy.

- Infection: it is possible that you could get an infection after the surgery. This can happen at the source of the incision if you do not take proper care of it afterward. The doctor will make sure that you know the right steps to take care of the incision so there are fewer issues.

For the most part, you will be able to avoid these issues if you follow the advice that your doctor gives you and you make sure to follow the dietary guidelines that are given with this kind of procedure. Overall, the gastric sleeve is considered very safe and will ensure that you can see some of the weight loss goals that you have been working so hard on.

Chapter 2: Questions to Ask Your Doctor

Before you go and decide to get the gastric sleeve, it is a good idea to talk to your doctor and ask as many questions as possible. This is the only way to ensure that you are getting the surgery because it is right for your needs, not because you have heard that it worked for other people. Some other questions that you may want to ask your doctor include:

How much weight will I likely lose?

It is good to talk to your doctor about how much weight you could possibly lose once you are done with the surgery. For most people, you will lose about sixty percent of your extra weight over a two-year timeframe, and most of it is going to come off during that first year. The amount of weight that you will lose over the long-term though is going to depend on a few other options, rather than on the procedure. You will also need to watch out how much and types of foods you eat and how much exercise you complete.

Many people think that the gastric sleeve is a miracle surgery that will take away all of their problems. It can do some wonderful things, but you still need to put in the work as well. If you don't eat well-portioned meals and you don't work out, you could gain all of your weight back.

Is it possible for my stomach to stretch when surgery is done?

It is possible for the stomach to stretch, but this is going to depend on how much you eat. If you have a large meal on occasion, it is possible that the stomach will try to stretch out to accommodate this, but then it will go back to the smaller size. However, if you continue to eat large meals all the time, then it will continue to stretch out and you will not be able to get it back. If you end up stretching out the stomach, you will start to eat more food again and gain thereby gaining back the weight.

When you get this kind of surgery, it is important that you learn how to monitor the amount of food that you are eating. Even having a small sweet on occasion is better than eating too much of what is considered healthy food because at least you aren't making the stomach stretch back out.

Can I have any alcohol?

While you shouldn't consume alcohol right after surgery while you are recovering, it is possible to have some. Remember that drinking alcohol now is going to make you feel drunk much faster, which is why some people choose to avoid it at all. You may not be used to how much alcohol will affect you. Studies have shown that those who have never had an issue with alcohol abuse can become alcoholics and get DWIs within two years of their surgery because they may be drinking the same amount that they did before and they don't realize how much this is going to affect them.

In addition to worrying about the toxicity of alcohol to you now that you finished the surgery, it is important to remember that alcohol is a carb with lots of calories. You want to keep your calorie count down as low as possible to help you maintain your weight loss, so take that into consideration before you choose to drink.

Will I have any sensitivities from this surgery?

It is more likely that you will have a higher sensitivity to proteins and carbs as well as to some of the vitamins and minerals that you take in once you are done with the surgery. Some people claim that they also become more sensitive to the smells around them. You will have to take things slowly when the surgery is done to see what things seem to bother you the most.

Will I experience a lot of pain?

This one is hard to answer because each person is going to experience pain in a different way. Open surgery can be pretty painful and you will end up spending more time in the hospital compared to doing laparoscopic surgery. Often the biggest amount of pain is going to come from the incision site, which is part of why the open surgery is going to hurt more. If you are good about following the dietary guidelines that are given to patients before surgery and you work to make the liver a bit smaller, it is easier for the surgeon to perform surgery that will be less painful. Luckily, the pain is easily managed during the beginning with some pain medications.

On the first day, you will not have too much pain, although you may be a bit groggy because of the medications that you are taking. The area of the incision is going to be sore and some people will feel a bit nauseated because of the anesthesia. During the first day, the surgeon will have you get up and walk around a bit because it can reduce some of your pain. It will be a bit difficult to do this, but it is much better than just sitting still.

The next day, you will start to notice the pain more than on the first day, mostly because the anesthesia has started to wear off a bit. You will still be given some pain medication and you will be required to move around more than the previous day. You will also switch over to the oral medication rather than the IV medication. You may notice that your throat is sore and dry from the anesthesia, but some water will be able to help with this. You will complete a swallow test during this day and you will be tested to see if you are able to get up and move around.

For the next few days, you will notice that you are experiencing the most amount of pain, mostly because you will be up and moving more often compared to what you did while in the hospital. Your doctor will make sure that you have the right instructions for how to manage your pain during this time, but make sure that you let them know if the pain gets to be too much.

After you get through the first week or so, you should notice that life is going to start getting back to normal. The pain will sometimes flare up, but for the most part, you will not feel it all that much. You still should avoid returning to work during this time even if the pain is not too bad. You need to give your body some time to recover first. By the time you get past the second week, you really should not be feeling pain at all. You will probably be able to get off your pain medication and can get back to your regular routine.

What is stomach stapling?

With this procedure, your stomach is going to be stapled together with a surgical staple gun when the surgeon does either a gastric bypass or a gastric sleeve procedure. The staples will close in the shape of a B to both compressed enough to not let the stomach bleed but still allowing your blood flow to get through. This allows the tissue to heal properly since it still gets some blood flow. These staples are going to stay in forever because they are made out of titanium. Even if they end up moving a bit out of their original position, they aren't going to cause any problems for you.

How much does this surgery cost?

There are going to be some costs that are associated with this kind of surgery and there will be some costs after the surgery that will stick with you for the rest of your life. The price for a nutritionist is going to be negotiated before you visit, but it will usually cost you between $50 and $100 each visit and you will need to pay for these out of pocket. You will also need to purchase the right foods, protein powders, and different size clothing for when you lose weight.

The cost of one of these sleeves is going to cost less than doing a gastric bypass, but a bit more compared to getting the gastric band surgery. The costs will usually range between $9,600 and $26,000 depending on where you get the surgery done. You will also need to have some follow-up visits with the surgery, which will be free, but if complications come up, you will have to pay to treat these.

Is this a permanent solution?

The gastric sleeve is designed to be a tool to help you get to your weight loss goals. It is meant to help you out when most of the other solutions just are not helping you lose enough weight or there are some serious issues with your health and you need to lose weight quickly. It can be a permanent solution, but it is going to depend a lot on the work that you do.

If you go into this surgery thinking that it is going to solve all of your problems, that you will not need to do anything else and you refuse to change your diet or activity level, you are going to be disappointed. It is possible for your stomach to stretch back out after the surgery, which will cause you to gain back any of the weight that you lost.

On the other hand, if you go into this with realistic expectations and you realize that you have to put in some effort with your activity level and diet, it can be a long-term solution for weight loss. You can work with your nutritionist to help you understand the meals that you should have to keep your weight down while still getting the nutrients that the body needs.

Why do I have to work with a nutritionist?

Before you decide to go through with this kind of surgery, you will need to make sure that you pick out the nutritionist that you want to work with. This nutritionist may seem like an extra cost and that it is just there to take up more of your time, but they are really going to make a difference in how much weight you will be able to lose.

You will be surprised at how different things will be when you are done with the surgery. Your stomach is going to be smaller so you will have to take in smaller portions and you will feel full much faster than before. You will have to concentrate on the nutrient density inside of your favorite foods to ensure that you are getting what the body needs, rather than just eating whatever you want. Even the amount of liquids that you consume, especially the times that you drink, will matter. Your nutritionist will be able to help you get through some of these obstacles so you can lose a lot of weight and feel better.

It is important to ask a lot of questions before you decide to get started with the gastric sleeve. This is a serious surgery that is going to cause some pain, will require you to make some lifestyle changes and will cost money. Understanding everything that goes into this surgery is important before you decide to jump in and give it a try.

Chapter 3: Your Diet Before Surgery

It is important that you understand what this kind of surgery entails. You not only have to worry about the surgery, but you have to be careful to make sure that you are following the right instructions even before you get to the operating room. Some people think that this gastric sleeve is a miracle treatment and that they are able to continue with the same dietary habits that they are used to. But your new diet guidelines are going to start before you get the operation done.

Some people believe that they are able to binge eat and enjoy whatever they want right up until they get to their operation day, but they are wrong. You need to make sure that you are following a strict diet for at least a few weeks ahead of time. Your surgeon will tell you the requirements that you need to follow before surgery and it is up to you to keep with it.

Since you are already obese when you want to be able to lose weight with the gastric sleeve, it is likely that your liver is full of fat. In order for the surgeon to access your stomach in this operation, they will need to be able to move aside the liver. If the liver is full of fat, it is going to still be hard for the surgeon to get to your stomach and perform the operation, and sometimes they will decide to cancel the operation because they just can't get to it.

By working on a stringent diet, you are ensuring that the doctor will be able to do a laparoscopic procedure, which is a lot easier and quicker to complete. This helps to keep the pain down and makes it so that the doctor can get the work done. But for this to work, you need to make sure that you stick with the diet plan, or it is all going to fail.

The requirements

There are going to be quite a few requirements that happen when you want to get a gastric sleeve. First, you will be required to increase the amount of protein that you are consuming so up the protein powders and lean meats. At the same time, you do need to start lowering your consumption of carbs by avoiding options like rice, cereal, pasta, and bread. And of course, you do need to make sure that you get rid of as many sugars as possible including soda, juices, desserts, and candy.

This is a great way to make sure that you are getting started on your new diet properly. You won't want to overeat once the sleeve is done, otherwise, you will stretch out the stomach again and the weight will come back. It is going to be hard in the beginning, but you will see that it makes things easier down the line.

Two weeks before surgery

You will need to make sure that you get started on this new diet at least two weeks before you are supposed to go into surgery. The earlier that you choose to go on the diet though, the better off you will be. The goal is to help you gain some of the healthy habits that your body needs once the sleeve is done, plus, it will help to get rid of some of the fat that is building up on your liver.

This is going to be the hardest part of the whole thing. For the most part, people who have gone on the gastric sleeve are the ones who are already obese and most likely don't have the best eating habits in place to start with. If you have been struggling with this kind of diet plan for some time now, it is fine to get started as early as possible. You aren't limited to just two weeks so if you would like to have a few extra weeks to help you out, that is just fine.

Remember that if you are not successful with going on this diet plan ahead of time, your doctor is going to postpone your surgery, which can add in a long wait and maybe, even more, expenses in the process. If you keep up with the bad eating habits, even if you do happen to get the surgery that you want, you will just end up gaining the weight back as the stomach stretches out again after the surgery.

This is why you will be required to talk to a nutritionist before, during, and after the surgery. They will be able to discuss some more of the exact nutrients that your body needs, such as how many calories you should stick with, how much protein and how many carbs you need, and so on. While it is important to eat foods that are full of healthy fats for energy and to keep your protein level high while your carb intake is as low as possible, you do need to make sure that you get more personalized help from your nutritionist.

Two days before surgery

Hopefully, at this point, you were already successful with the diet requirements that were set for you for the two weeks, or more, prior to the surgery. This is going to help limit the amount of fat that is found in the liver so that the surgery will go a little bit easier, and will ensure that you are already starting on some of the healthy habits that are needed for after the surgery.

However, once you get to the time period that is about two days before the surgery there will be a few other requirements and restrictions that you need to follow. In addition to the requirements that you were following in the two weeks before surgery, you will also need to follow these diet rules:

- Omit any beverage that is carbonated
- Omit caffeine
- Change your diet to one that is of clear liquids so that you will be able to get through the surgery. This would include options like water, Jell-O, sugar-free popsicles, and broth. It is sometimes fine to drink a protein shake each day to help keep your levels of energy up, but you will need to discuss this one with your nutritionist to see if it is allowed. It is important to stay off sugars during this time.

- Follow any of the other instructions that your surgeon gives for your specific case.

The last two days before you have surgery can be really restrictive, but these are often general rules for any surgery to make sure that your stomach is not incredibly full when it is time to have the surgery. Your doctor will be able to answer any questions that you have about this diet plan and they may also choose to give you some extra advice as well, if needed.

Chapter 4: The Day of Surgery

Congratulations! You have made it to this point and now it is time to get ready for the surgery! Your work is not done. Sure, you have spent some time changing up your diet plan in the hopes of living a healthier lifestyle so that the gastric sleeve will help more than ever, but now it is time for the part where you are going to learn the diet you will need for the day of the surgery, and for afterwards. You will not be able to go back to eating as much as you want and your past eating habits and still maintain the weight loss that you want.

For the first few weeks after your surgery, your diet will be a little bit different. The point of this diet is to make sure that you reduce the risks that you can experience after the surgery. It may seem a little bit overly cautious, but you will need to spend some time consuming just clear liquids and you will need to stick with the diet very closely. Some patients think that they are feeling fine and they should be able to go back to normal eating patterns, but unless the doctor says it is fine, do not try to do that.

If you end up cheating on this post-op diet, you are going to suffer from some serious issues. You could cause a gastric leak, which is when the food you eat ends up getting through the line of staples and goes into the abdomen. If this ends up happening while you are still in the hospital, the doctor can go back and do another surgery to flush out the system. But if this ends up happening, later on, it could become a life-threatening infection. You could also end up with bowel obstruction, diarrhea, and constipation.

You will be able to add in some regular food later on (you won't be stuck on a liquid diet for the rest of your life), but you do need to do so in the right manner to make sure that you aren't causing harm in your body.

After the surgery is done, you will feel some pain, so it will cause some irritability during that time. This can make it hard for some people to eat at all and you may not want to eat anything. You should still try to get a little bit into your body to ensure that you get the nutrients you need to heal after surgery, but you don't want to overdo it.

On the day of the surgery, you may notice that you are thirsty when the operation is all done. You will be told that you can't have anything to drink or eat until the day after the surgery. The breathing tubs that you have in your throat will make it hard and unpleasant anyway. Depending on the surgeon, you may be allowed to have a bit of ice or some mouth swabs to help out.

The day after your surgery, you are going to meet with your radiologist. They are going to give you a swallow test, which is meant to test whether there will be any major leaks in the stomach before you are given water. You are given a bit more freedom on this day, but you will still be required to keep it all down to a minimum.

You are still not allowed to have any caffeine or carbonated drinks during this day. These kinds of drinks will create what is known as a diuretic effect and it is the main reason that those patients who end up cheating and drinking a beverage that has caffeine are readmitted because of dehydration.

Your friends and family may decide to come and visit you in the hospital during this time. You need to make sure that you are not accepting food or drinks from these people, no matter how well-intentioned they may be. You will be given a list of foods that are allowed and those that are not and if the food is on the not allowed list, no matter how good it may smell at the time, you should not consume it. There is a reason that your doctor doesn't want you to consume some foods, so make sure to follow their advice.

It is likely that on this first day you are still going to be thirsty. You will be told to stay with mostly water and you will need to drink it slowly to make sure you are not causing any issues with your stomach. If you are feeling it, you may be able to have a little something else including strained cream soup, sugar-free gelatin, broth, unsweetened juice, and milk.

During those first few days, you will not want to spend your time eating a lot of food and it is likely that your doctor will keep you mostly limited to just clear liquids, like water, for the first bit to keep things gentle on your stomach. As you will see in the next chapter, you will slowly be able to add in some solid foods back to your diet, but it will take some time and it is likely that you will find you have a few food sensitivities in the process.

Chapter 5: Your Diet After the Surgery

After a few days, you will be sent home and will have to stick to the diet that your surgeon gives you. This chapter is going to look at some of the guidelines for the first bit after your surgery, but remember that your surgeon may give you some specific guidelines that you are able to follow that is unique for your situation. Make sure that you follow those recommendations as closely as possible. They may seem a little bit restrictive, but they are there to allow your stomach to heal and to ensure that you don't run into other problems later on.

Now we are going to move on to day two and three after the surgery. You are more likely to be on your own at this time since your partner and others around you may have headed back to work. Unless you have lined up some help (which can be a good idea since you will still be in a lot of pain), you will have to get everything that is needed.

The foods that you are allowed to eat for these days will be up to the surgeon. There are times when the surgeon will have you stay on a liquid diet until the week is up, but sometimes you will be allowed to have some pureed foods towards the end of the week.

If you have been given permission to have pureed food, you have to make sure that it is completely smooth and there are no lumps inside of it at this time, or it can cause some issues on the stomach. Some of the foods that your surgeon may allow in pureed form include lean ground meat, beans, fish, yogurt, and soft fruit. You will still have to keep your liquids to those like water, fat-free milk, juice, and broth.

Remember that during this time your body is still trying to get used to all of this fluid from food, but you should be getting mostly fluids rather than worrying about nutrients right now. If all you are able to handle is some water or broth for a few more days, that is just fine. Your desire for eating food is not going to be strong and most people during this time will not worry about even eating the pureed foods right now.

As we mentioned, you are not going to have a huge desire to eat food after your surgery. Ghrelin, or the hunger hormone, is not going to exist inside of you. This is mostly because the area where this hormone is made inside the stomach has been removed. Depending on how your surgery went and each individual person, you may stay on the liquid diet for just a few days or you could be on it for a week or more.

During this time, focus on nutrient dense foods if you are able to consume them You should not have any foods that are unhealthy for you so make sure to avoid things like carbonated beverages, sweet beverages, sugar, and caffeine. You are not going to feel like eating a lot of food at this time and any foods that you do eat need to have a lot of nutrients so that you can keep your energy up and get through recovery after the surgery.

Once you reach the second week, you are going to notice that your hunger levels will go up a little bit, but they will still be pretty low. You will probably still be on a mostly liquid diet at this point, but you could add in some options like protein shakes to help give your body more energy. Hopefully, you spent some time testing out different protein shakes before the surgery so you know what you will like the most and can add in one of these each day to help.

Your surgeon and your nutritionist will be able to give you some more advice on how much you are able to eat so that you don't harm your stomach but you are still getting something in there. But for the most part, some of the things that you will be allowed to eat include:

- Protein powder: you need to make sure that this is mixed with some kind of clear liquid that doesn't have carbonation and is sugar-free, like water
- Creamed soups that don't have any chunks inside
- Soups with some soft noodles
- Sugar-free sorbet
- Non-fat yogurt
- Watery oatmeal with no sugar

- Yogurt
- Pudding
- Thinned applesauce, but do not add in sugar to this

By the time you get to week three, it is time to start adding in some more normal food to the diet. But be cautious though because it is likely that you are going to feel a little bit sick when you eat them. Some of the foods are going to taste a bit different to you and your stomach may not tolerate some old favorites as well. For example, some people find that after this surgery they end up having an intolerance to dairy. It is best to introduce new foods one by one. That way, if something causes you some issue, you will know which one to avoid for awhile. Make sure that you keep track of the foods that offend you and how it bothered you so that you can keep track of this for later.

You will also want to make sure that during this time you continue to keep your fat and sugar intake to a minimum. This will make sure that you don't irritate the stomach or take in more calories than you need. There are three main goals that you will need to work on each day including:

- Try to get as close to 60 grams of protein into your diet each day.
- Always eat your meals slowly. This will help to reduce some of the pain that you are feeling.

- Make sure that you introduce only one new food at a time and that they are never introduced during the same meal. This helps you to figure out which ones are giving you trouble.

While we are on this third week, you need to make sure that you avoid a few items that could cause you irritation. You have to avoid fibrous vegetables like leafy greens, asparagus, celery, and broccoli. Starchy foods like bread, rice, and pasta shouldn't be used either. Also, be careful with the amount of sugar that is found inside of your protein shakes. Sometimes the fruity ones will have a higher amount of sugar in them so you have to be careful.

The good news is that there are still a lot of choices that you can make when it comes to allowed foods during this week; just remember that you need to take it slowly. Some of the options available to you include:

- Scrambled eggs
- Soups
- Ground chicken with stock
- Ground beef with stock
- Steamed vegetables
- Soft or soggy cereal
- Soft cheese
- Cottage cheese as long as it is low in fat
- Hummus
- Coconut milk and almond milk in your shakes

- One protein shake each day
- Mashed avocados
- Mashed fruit
- Canned salmon or tuna

Make sure that you take things slowly so that you don't end up irritating your stomach so much during this time and so you can catch any of the sensitivities that end up bothering you. This is not the time for you to start stuffing yourself and you will not even be able to get back to normal eating habits yet, but you are building up to it.

And when you get to week four, you are able to finally introduce some real food into your diet. You can't go completely back yet, partly because you have been used to such an easy diet that it is hard to go straight back, but eating some soft versions of your old food options, and eating slowly, will allow you to get back to a somewhat normal eating habit.

You do have to remember that your stomach is still going to be sensitive during this time and there are a few foods that you need to avoid at this time to keep the sensitivities away. You need to avoid some options like whole milk, high carb foods like pasta and bread, nuts, fried foods, desserts, candy, sugary drinks, dairy foods that are whole fat, and sodas.

This is the time when you will be able to add back in a lot of the healthy foods that you want, as long as you keep your portions small. Beef and chicken are fine to eat as long as you eat them slowly and keep them soft. Soft potatoes, vegetables, fruits, and cereal are fine as well. And don't forget to go with your protein shakes each day so that you can get that added nutrition that is needed but may still be hard to get at this time.

In some cases, your surgeon will allow you to start having a few small snacks in between meals at this time, depending on how well your surgery is healing. This would need to be a small snack of hundred calories or so, but can help you get on a better eating schedule and can help with some of the hunger that may have started coming back. For example, having one hard-boiled egg, a quarter cup of oatmeal, or some fresh fruit is often allowed for snacking.

Once you get past the first month, you will have some more freedom in the foods that you are allowed to eat. You can pretty much go back to eating most foods, but your portions should be a lot smaller to help prevent stretching out of the stomach. Continue to just add in one food at a time and then take note of how you feel so you can tell if you have an intolerance to that food. Your doctor will officially clear you sometimes between five weeks and three months to start eating solid foods again.

Guidelines for every state

We talked in some detail about the different requirements for eating during the different weeks after surgery. Your doctor will give you some specific recommendations based on your personal history and how the stomach is healing. No matter how you are doing though, there are a few guidelines that you can always follow to ensure that you are seeing weight loss, that you are getting the nutrients that are needed for recovery, and that you aren't causing any harm to the healing stomach. Some of these guidelines include:

- Eat three smaller meals during the day. You may be surprised at how small you will need to keep the meals as you are healing. Your protein intake should be the most important.
- Get your fluids. You want to get in plenty, but make sure that you don't drink anything for at least 30 minutes before each meal. This will help you have room for the meal.
- Try to keep snacks to a minimum and don't add them in until at least a few weeks after surgery. When eating your snacks, go for fruits and veggies.
- Take a multivitamin during this time. Especially in those first few weeks, you will not have much of an appetite so that vitamin can help you stay healthy.
- Go for about 60 grams of protein each day. Your protein shake will really help with this.

- Try to get in a little bit of exercise each day, once it has been approved by the doctor.
- Always make sure that you avoid sodas, although, by the time you get past the first month, you can add in a bit of caffeine from coffee or tea.
- Learn coping mechanisms for those days that end up being a little tough. Having an accountability partner can really help out.

Getting past the three months

By the time you finish up with three months post-surgery, you should notice that you lost quite a bit of weight. This is mostly because you didn't eat nearly as much as you are used to before, some of that during the few weeks when food just irritated you. Sometime after the three months, your doctor will allow you to eat some solid foods, and you should notice that you will feel full much faster when you eat than before. Make sure that at every meal, you chew your foods well and eat slowly.

During this stage, you will still need to meet with your dietician to help you out in the future. You are probably very happy with your weight loss results so far with this surgery, but you have to keep up with it in order to not stretch the stomach out and gain all of the weight back. With some hard work and sticking with the diet, you are going to see some of the results stick around and can still see a lot of weight loss, even past the three-month mark.

As you can see, there are some strict rules when it comes to what you are allowed to eat after having gastric sleeve surgery. Following these guidelines, as well as any of the guidelines that your doctor gives to you, are critical to ensuring that the surgery goes well. This is not just about helping you lose weight, even though you will lose some weight with this program, but it is about helping you to keep safe after going through a major surgery.

Chapter 6: Stomach Stretching After Surgery

Besides being able to get rid of the hunger hormone in the stomach, the other purpose of going through the gastric sleeve surgery is to shrink up the size of your stomach so that you will eat less. But one question that some people who are considering this type of surgery will ask is whether the stomach is able to stretch back out again over time. There is a lot of time, pain, and money that goes into this kind of surgery, and people are interested to know how successful the surgery can be.

There is a possibility that you will be able to stretch out your stomach again after the surgery, but whether or not this is going to occur, along with the weight that comes with a stretched-out stomach, is going to depend on the patient. The surgery will help to get rid of the majority of your hunger hormones and can make your stomach way smaller, so you do have a big advantage in keeping weight off compared to other people. Theoretically, this advantage should stick around for the rest of the patient's life, however, the patient is the one who gets to make the decision and they get to decide if they want to put in the work to keep their stomach small.

A big factor in whether the patient will be able to keep off the weight gain and keep their stomach from stretching is whether they are successful in their new exercise routine and diet plan, which they should design with the help of their nutritionist. Even with a small stomach, consuming just high-fat foods and sugary snacks will pack on the pounds. This surgery is not meant to be a quick fix; it is more like a tool that will help the patient work towards their specific weight loss goals. If the patient goes back to their old bad eating habits, they will most likely fail.

Fullness and hunger signals get messed up

So, to understand how this is going to work, let's take a look at the process of the stomach. The walls of your stomach will have folds of tissues that are trained to contract and expand in response to the food that comes into and leaves the stomach. Once the stomach has expanded out far enough, a signal is going to get to the brain that tells it that the stomach is full.

Acid is going to break down the food that you eat as soon as it enters the stomach. The stomach walls are going to get to work, contracting to push your food into the intestines so it can be digested even more. If you end up overeating on a regular basis, you will stretch the walls too many times, and the stomach is going to tell the brain that it is full at a much later time than it should. It can also still send out signals of hunger to the brain, even when food is still present in the stomach.

This broken signal system is one of the main reasons that people will eat more food than they should on a regular basis. When you keep eating more food because you think that you are still hungry, you are going to find that it becomes really difficult to lose weight.

Risks of stretching out stomach after surgery

As we mentioned before, it is possible to stretch out your stomach, even after the sleeve is performed. This is why you really do need to be careful about your diet and exercise routine after the surgery is completed, rather than just going back to some of your old ways of doing things and hoping it will all be fine. The gastric sleeve is supposed to be all about having the right tools to make the changes you need for weight loss, not hoping that the weight loss is going to magically happen without any changes from you.

There are a few things that can happen when you stretch out your stomach again after the operation. The most common issue is that you will start to gain weight again. You can, over time and if you eat a lot of bigger meals, stretch the stomach out so that it ends up as big as it was before. If you are back to the same size stomach and still eating these big meals, it is really hard to keep the weight off, even with the stitches in place.

These stitches are meant to help make your stomach smaller and they can be really effective at getting this done. But your stomach muscles are also stretchable so you need to be careful with listening to your hunger and fullness cues and only eating as much as you need. Of course, if you have one big meal on occasion, it is not going to be the end of the world. But you do need to watch out for how often you are eating and to make sure that your portions stay where they need.

There could be some more serious complications based on how small your surgeon made the stomach and how quickly you end up stretching it out after the surgery is done. If you are not very good about sticking with your diet and go back to your former ways of eating before fully recovering, or soon after recovery, you could end up with some issues.

Stretching the stomach too fast could end up with some serious conditions such as bleeding, tearing in the stomach, and even stomach leaking. Your doctor will check for some of these issues before you leave the hospital so if something went wrong with the surgery, they are able to fix it as soon as possible. With that said, if you are eating foods that are too heavy on the body, that you have sensitivities to, or will irritate the stomach or you are eating too much food on a regular basis, these could be serious health concerns that you have to deal with after your operation.

To make sure that you are not dealing with any of these adverse side effects, you need to be careful with what you eat. If you struggled with eating before you got this surgery and you are hoping that this surgery will be a miracle fix that does all of the work, you are more likely to put yourself at risk. Learning how to eat right and the right portion sizes for you, which your nutritionist can help you out with, will make a world of difference.

Chapter 7: Strategies to See Long-Term Success

One misconception that comes with getting the gastric sleeve surgery is that it will do all of the work and it will last forever. It is true that it can help you to lose a lot of weight quickly, but you are still responsible for putting in the work and making sure that the weight loss actually sticks around. If you get through the recovery phase and then go right back to your old habits, you will see that the weight will come right back, even with a smaller stomach.

For many who get this kind of surgery, it is important that you develop some healthy eating habits and start up with a new active lifestyle if you would like to see the weight loss results that you are promised with this surgery. This chapter is going to help you out by providing you with some of the best strategies for long-term success with the gastric sleep surgery.

Use tricks to keep yourself on track

Eating a big meal on occasion, such as having one on Thanksgiving, is not going to mess up your signals all that bad, but doing it all of the time will stretch out your stomach and will end up causing some issues with the signals. Once you are done with your gastric sleeve surgery, you will want to make sure that the stretching out does not occur again, or you can end up losing out on all that pain and money.

The good news is that there are a few things that you are able to do to make sure that you keep your stomach small when the surgery is done. These tasks include:

When you are done with your surgery, you will need to limit the amount of sugar in your diet (pretty much to just a little bit in fruit and the little bit in your protein shakes), to help you during the recovery. Even as you progress later in time, after the recovery process is over and you are able to eat more solid foods, you will have to be careful with the amount of sugar that you consume. This can be hard for most people, so why not consider giving yourself a small reward each week. It needs to be a small treat, but there is nothing wrong with having a little something sweet, as long as it is on occasion. It is much better to have that little treat than to overeat or overindulge later on.

The next thing that you can work on is to not drink when you eat. Your stomach is going to be a lot smaller so if you drink too much, you will either end up causing the stomach to stretch or you won't eat as much because the stomach is already full. It is best to drink the fluids that you need about an hour or two before and after you eat, so that you can get the healthy nutrients that your body needs, and which can be harder for the body to get once your stomach is smaller.

While it is fine to have an occasional large meal, such as at Thanksgiving, make sure that you do not go crazy with this one. Your next few meals should be small to help you stay with the new healthy habits that you are on. You do not want to allow those large meals to become a habit and then risk stretching out your stomach.

If you are sticking with your small meals and drinking plenty of fluids, but still finds that you are feeling hungry, it is fine to eat a very small snack in between the small meals that you are having. Almonds are a good choice as are healthy fruits and vegetables. If you need some ideas for healthy snacks, or even for some healthy meals, go out and look for a recipe book that is meant to help patients who have gotten gastric sleeves.

In some cases, you may end up going off track. You may overeat a few times and feel bad about it. No matter how badly you messed up, get back on track as soon as possible. It is important to not become discouraged at all. If you find that you are still having a lot of trouble limiting the portions you should be eating, it is time to give your surgeon a call.

Learn how to control your portion sizes

One of the hardest things that you will have to learn about when you are done with your gastric sleeve surgery is how to control your portion sizes. We live in a country where portion sizes are huge and even if you think that you are doing a good job keeping the portions down, you will probably be surprised at how many calories you are consuming.

If you want to keep the weight loss off, you have to take control over your own portions. This is sometimes difficult if you end up going to a restaurant or if you are eating at someone else's home where you are going to be a little bit more limited on how big the serving sizes are. At home, you can weigh and measure the food to make sure that it fits the needs that you have. When you eat somewhere else, this is not really an option. Some of the ways that you can take more control over your portion size when you eat out at a restaurant include:

- When you receive your meal, get a box and place half of the meal inside. Then you can sit back and enjoy the half that you have in front of you.
- If you end up going out to eat with someone else, consider splitting the meal with them. This makes it easier to eat less because both of you will be eating it.

- If it is available, see if the restaurant will give you a lunch size of the meal. These are usually a lot smaller so they won't pack on as many calories.
- Instead of ordering one of the full meals at the restaurant, consider going with an appetizer or a few side dishes to help you stay on track.

There are some situations where you will be a guest at someone's home and they may be in charge of the portions that you are getting. It is just fine to tell them that you only want a certain amount put on your plate. If it ends up being too much, it is fine for you to leave some of it on your plate and let them know that the meal was delicious, but that you are just too full to finish.

Know your triggers

Every person who has ever struggled with weight loss knows that there is something that sets them off and makes it hard to stay on their best-laid plans. It is important to realize that just because you are getting this surgery doesn't mean that you will never have to deal with that trigger again. You have to find a healthy way to deal with the trigger, whether it is eating a little bit of sugar sets you off to eating too much or you overeat when you are sad or stressed out from work.

There are a lot of healthy ways that you can deal with these triggers, you just need to learn to find the one that works for you. It is fine to indulge sometimes, but if you let the triggers get in the way, even the gastric sleeve is not going to be able to help you out.

Plan ahead

Planning ahead is going to be one of your best allies when it comes to keeping the weight loss off. There will be times when you really crave something sweet when you don't have the most time to make a meal that night, or something else comes up. You have to be the one in control of the situation, otherwise, you are going to end up failing.

The good news is that there are a few ways that you can plan ahead. The first idea is to keep some healthy snacks around. While your appetite is going to go way down when you have the operation done, there will still be some times when you get really hungry in between your small meals, especially if you are pretty active. Instead of reaching for a cookie or one of those other unhealthy snacks, planning ahead and keeping some fruits and vegetables around can make a big difference.

This doesn't mean that you are never allowed to have a little something sweet. In fact, completely preventing yourself from having these snacks can make it difficult for you to stay on the diet plan. Keeping a few guilty pleasure snacks around in single servings can help you on those few times you would like to cheat.

Add in some exercise

While the gastric sleeve is going to do some wonders for helping you to lose some weight on your own since you are cutting down on the amount of food that you consume and trying to eat healthier, it is important to start in on a healthy exercise routine as well. This exercise routine is so important because it helps to tone the body, lifts up your mood, and will make it easier to lose and keep off that weight.

This does not mean that you have to be obsessed with working out to see the results. You just need to be careful with not sitting still all day and eating. Getting out for a nice walk, going to the gym a few times a week, or finding some other way to be more active will be just fine.

The first few weeks after you are done with the surgery, you will most likely just need to sit back and relax. You do not want to cause more harm to the surgery area and you will most likely be in a lot of pain from it as well. But as soon as you receive the all-clear from your doctor, it is just fine to get out there and do some light exercise. Over time, you can build up to some more moderate levels as well.

The gastric sleeve can be a great resource to make sure that you lose weight and keep it off, especially for those who have had a lot of trouble doing this in the past. But you have to actively work to keep your stomach smaller and to lose the weight. The gastric sleeve can do this for you temporarily, but if you do not change up some of your own bad habits, you will never see the weight loss stick around.

Conclusion

Thanks for making it through to the end of this book, let's hope it was informative and able to provide you with all of the tools you need to achieve your goals whatever they may be.

The next step is to talk to your doctor if you feel that the gastric sleeve is the right choice for you. This is a serious surgery and not one to take lightly. Those who only want to lose a few pounds, or those who are trying to lose weight quickly without making any changes to their personal habits and diets, will find that this is not the choice for them. Only you and your doctor are able to decide if the gastric sleeve is right for you and if you are ready to make the changes that are necessary.

This guidebook took some time to talk about the gastric sleeve and some of the things that you will encounter with this surgery. We talked about what the gastric sleeve was, some of the benefits of going with this operation, and how it compares to some of the other options that are out there. In addition, we talked about the different diets that you will need to be on during this process, including before, during, and after the surgery. It is important for you to understand everything that goes into this kind of surgery, and this guidebook aims to answer some of your pressing questions.

If you are struggling with losing weight and have considered working with the gastric sleeve, take some time to read through this guidebook to learn what you need to know to prepare for this operation.

Finally, if you found this book useful in any way, a review on Amazon is always appreciated!

www.ingramcontent.com/pod-product-compliance
Lightning Source LLC
Chambersburg PA
CBHW060807260726
48660CB00002B/828